Writing Practice
For Doctors

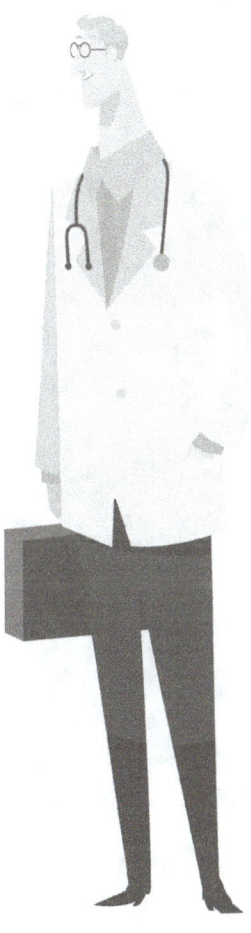

ISBN: 9781677230952
Copyright © 2019 Tim Bird.

All rights reserved. No part of this publication may be reproduced, distributed, or transmitted in any form or by any means, including photocopying, recording, or other electronic or mechanical methods, without the prior written permission of the publisher.

The contents of this book are believed to be correct at time of printing. Nevertheless the publisher cannot accept responsibility for errors and omissions, changes in the detail given or for any expense or loss thereby caused.

Technique

1. Rest the pen on your middle finger: A. and the area between your index finger and thumb: B.

2. Pinch the end of the pen/pencil with your index finger: C. and thumb: D.

3. Relax your hand and follow the arrows to trace the letter.

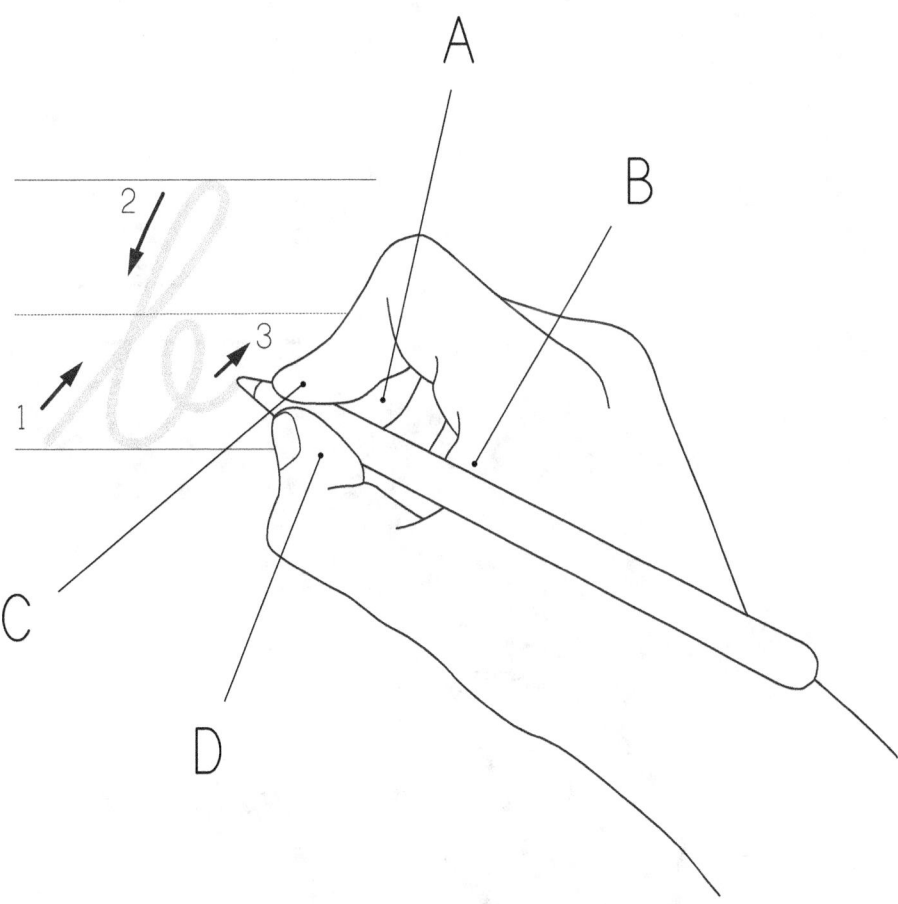

R_X PRESCRIPTION

Apple

a a

a a a a a

a a a a a

a a a a a

a a a a a

a a a a a

a a a a a

R_X PRESCRIPTION

Bed Rest

$\mathcal{B}$ $\textit{b}$

PRESCRIPTION

Counselling

C c

PRESCRIPTION

Diamorphine

D d

R_X PRESCRIPTION

Exercise

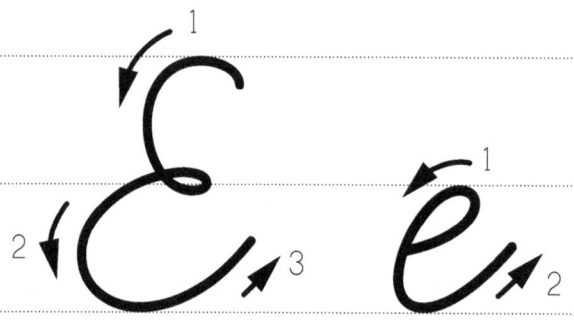

Rx PRESCRIPTION

Fat Farm

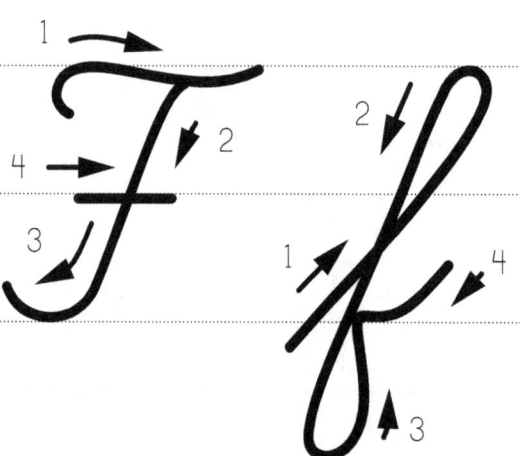

Rx PRESCRIPTION

Gastric Bypass

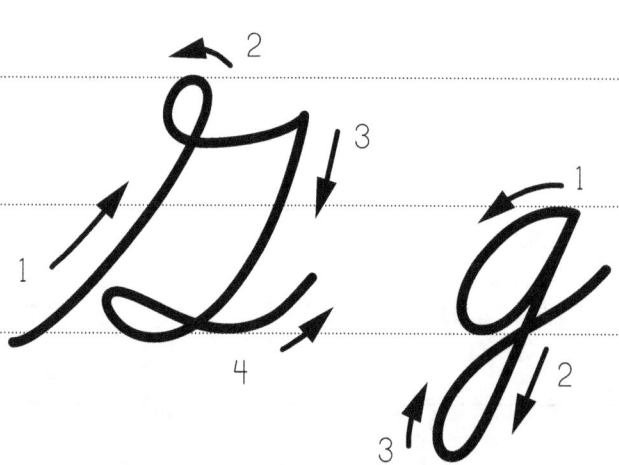

Rx PRESCRIPTION

Hangover Cure

___
___

H h

Rx PRESCRIPTION

Iron Pills

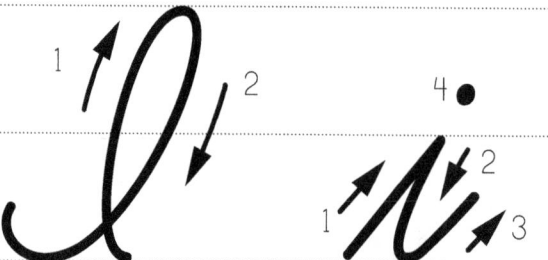

Rx PRESCRIPTION

Juice Diet

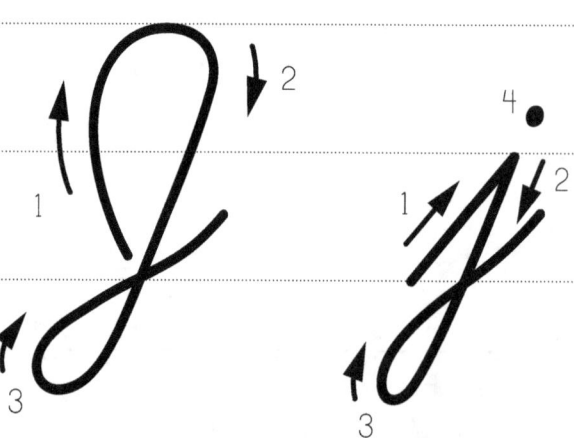

Rx PRESCRIPTION

Knee Replacement

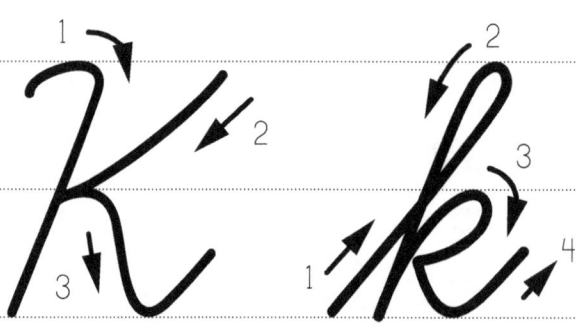

Rx PRESCRIPTION

Laxatives

$\mathcal{L}\ \mathit{l}$

Rx PRESCRIPTION

Malaria Tablets

M m

m m m m m

m m m m m

m m m m m

m m m m m

m m m m m

m m m m m

R̽ PRESCRIPTION

Nasal Spray

_____
_____
_____

N m

RX PRESCRIPTION

Osteopath

𝒪 𝒪

R̲X̲ PRESCRIPTION

Painkillers

P p

p *p* *p* *p* *p*

p *p* *p* *p* *p*

p *p* *p* *p* *p*

p *p* *p* *p* *p*

p *p* *p* *p* *p*

p *p* *p* *p* *p*

R̲X̲ PRESCRIPTION

Quit Smoking

Q q

℞ PRESCRIPTION

Relaxation

R r

Rx PRESCRIPTION

Sleeping Pills

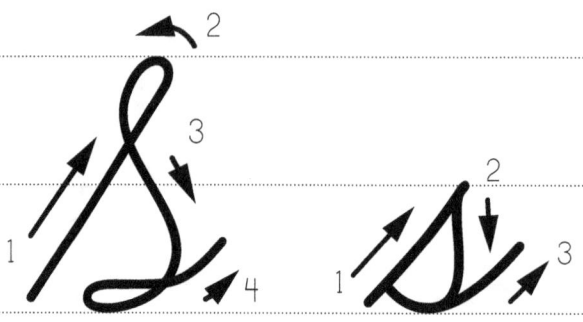

R̆x PRESCRIPTION

Therapy

R_X PRESCRIPTION

Ultrasound Scan

u u u u u

u u u u u

u u u u u

u u u u u

u u u u u

R_X PRESCRIPTION

Vitamins

R_X PRESCRIPTION

Weight Loss

W w

R̲x̲ PRESCRIPTION

X - Ray

R_X PRESCRIPTION

Yoga

Y y

Y Y Y Y Y

Y Y Y Y Y

Y Y Y Y Y

Y Y Y Y Y

Y Y Y Y Y

Y Y Y Y Y

Rx PRESCRIPTION

Zinc Tablets

Did you like this book?

If you did then would you please consider leaving me some positive feedback on Amazon? It will help so much and allow me to continue making more books like this one.

Thank you!

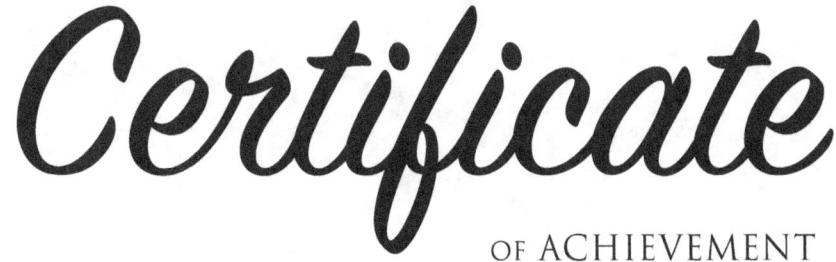

Certificate
OF ACHIEVEMENT

THIS CERTIFICATE IS PROUDLY PRESENTED TO

FOR MASTERING YOUR 'CURSIVE STYLE' ABC

Congratulations on completing the Writing Practice for Doctors book!

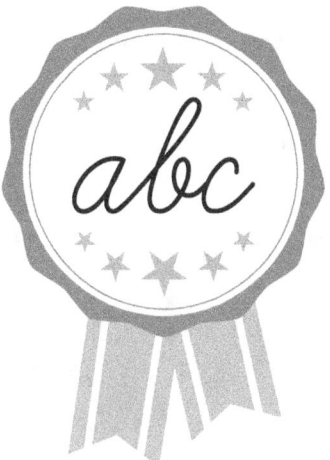

SIGNATURE   DATE

www.ingramcontent.com/pod-product-compliance
Lightning Source LLC
Chambersburg PA
CBHW080555220526
45466CB00010B/3160